Paula McLaren's Top Tips

When dealing with

a breast cancer diagnosis

Paula McLaren asserts the moral right to be identified as the author of this work.

All rights reserved. No part of this book may be reproduced, stored in a retrieval system, or transmitted, in any form or by any means, without the prior permission in writing of the author.

This book is designed to provide competent and reliable information regarding the subject matter covered. However, it is sold with the understanding that the author is not engaged in rendering professional or medical advice. If expert assistance is required, the services of a professional should be sought. The author will not be responsible for any losses or damages of any kind incurred by the reader whether indirectly or directly arising from the use of the information found in this book.

This book may not be re-sold and is only available in this form and may not be circulated in any form of binding or cover other than that in which it is published. If you have acquired this book from any other means you have an illegal copy.

No guarantees are made or implied. The reader assumes responsibility for use of information contained herein.

Copyright © 2014 Paula McLaren

All rights reserved.

ISBN: 1507526733
ISBN-13: 978-1507526736

ABOUT THE AUTHOR

Born with a keen sense of adventure, Paula McLaren aspired to travel the world from a young age, settling for many years in Orlando, Florida. Always living life to the full, experiencing travel industry work and qualifying as a Florida Realtor, Paula has made the most of every opportunity along the way.

After four years of living life back in the UK with her young son, Paula was diagnosed with early stage breast cancer in May 2011 after discovering a small lump in her right breast. Surgery, chemotherapy and radiotherapy followed.

Paula is now taking a break from a course of aromatase inhibitor treatment due to severe side effects, and has made many lifestyle changes including diet, exercise and reducing stress levels.

During Paula's cancer journey she experienced trials and tribulations with various aspects of the treatment. Making notes along the way to help her recovery Paula found she had acquired a great deal of information that could be of use to others in a similar situation.

This book was written unconsciously initially and if just one tip could help another person dealing with a breast cancer diagnosis then that is a great thing.

A portion of the book's proceeds will be donated to Macmillan and CHECT; both charities are very close to Paula's heart in different ways.

DEDICATION

For all those who have supported me with their love and kindness throughout, I am forever grateful... and for Sally Short and her incredible family, a true inspiration.

INDEX

	Foreword	
Tip 1	Wigs	1
Tip 2	Hats	6
Tip 3	Get Out Of The House	8
Tip 4	Support Team	9
Tip 5	Counselling	11
Tip 6	Websites	12
Tip 7	Breast Care Nurse	14
Tip 8	Hospital Appointments	16
Tip 9	Chemotherapy	20
Tip 10	Funny Films, Radio and Books	24
Tip 11	Children	26
Tip 12	Breast Cancer Support Groups	29
Tip 13	Positive Mental Attitude	30

Tip 14	Weight Loss	31
Tip 15	Alternative Therapies	33
Tip 16	Get Plenty Of Rest	34
Tip 17	Spoil Yourself Days	35
Tip 18	Keep A Diary	36
Tip 19	Relaxation Tapes, Meditation and Self-Hypnosis	37
Tip 20	How To Tell Your Family, Friends Or Complete Strangers	39
Tip 21	How To Deal With The Sudden Emotions	41
Tip 22	Radiotherapy	42
Tip 23	Drink Water	44
Tip 24	Be Grateful	45
Tip 25	Financial Challenges	46
Tip 26	Your Spouse/Partner	48
Tip 27	Hospital Stays During Treatment	49
Tip 28	Surgery	52
Tip 29	Decisions	54
Tip 30	When The Treatment Stops	55
Tip 31	How To Get Back To Normal	58
Tip 32	Tamoxifen And Endocrine Treatment	60

Tip 33	Aromatase Inhibitors	64
Tip 34	Bone Scan	66
Tip 35	Be Proactive Not Reactive	69
	Finally	72

FOREWORD

"There is a problem..."

When I was unlucky enough to hear the above words I suddenly found myself plunged onto the rollercoaster ride that immediately follows them. Whilst travelling through the daily highs and lows of further tests, discussions on how to proceed, ultrasounds, surgery, chemotherapy and radiotherapy I searched for anything that would help me deal with every aspect of this long road of treatment.

I found some wonderfully helpful books, many going into great detail. I had one experience of family cancer in the past and this also helped me when dealing with consultants, hospitals and the many decisions to be made.

During my journey of handling the daily unknown, I was introduced to someone through a mutual friend who was just starting her own journey after a breast cancer diagnosis. I was asked to chat over my experience so far and offer any helpful tips to get through the various stages I had encountered. A new friendship was formed and treasured over the coming months with the most amazing, courageous woman I could ever hope to meet.

An example was set and the fight was a hard one for my dear friend and as things gradually got worse I will always remember her words which never failed to be said. "Onwards and upwards" became the theme and her strength was passed on to me on a weekly, sometimes daily basis. As her battle was lost, I mourned my friend and admired the strength of her beautiful family. I will be forever grateful to have known such an incredible woman, a fine example of inner strength and courage.

After talking through a few of the stages I had encountered with Sally in the beginning, I realized I had picked up some tips that had I known them previously would have helped me a great deal. I kept a notepad full of affirmations, feelings, the challenges and how I had met each one. I felt relieved to be able to help someone else going through the uncertainty that I was. It occurred to me how useful I would have found it to have basic tips available to ease the process even slightly.

These are not in-depth, complicated points which could overwhelm someone already feeling that way.

The following tips are simply things that made a small difference and had I known them previously would have helped me face the challenges and possibly avoid some of the mistakes I made along the way. I wanted to share them with anyone else looking for help at such a traumatic time.

In any situation, I always think if you can take even one or two positive things which help at that time then that is a good thing.

You will not find detailed discussions in this book; there are already many useful books for that purpose. This is a book that is quick to read, simple to understand and was written by someone who knows the challenges of a breast cancer diagnosis. It offers tips to help with keeping your spirits up and get you through the stress of dealing with the unknown, which is where a cancer diagnosis leaves you.

I have left a few blank pages in the back of this book so you can make notes, start a diary of your journey, write down your thoughts or use in any way that will help.

A percentage of the profits from this book will be donated to Macmillan and CHECT.

Thank you for reading and I wish you all the very best of every single day.

In no particular order...

TIP 1
WIGS

As if it's not enough to be faced with a cancer diagnosis, there is also the traumatic realization that hair loss will most likely be inevitable if chemotherapy is a possible treatment.

I asked this question about hair loss immediately after my diagnosis and was told not to worry about it at that point, fantastic I thought. I then enquired again that same day when I was taken to talk to a breast care nurse a while later. The nurse confirmed that it would indeed most likely be the case that I would have chemotherapy and lose my hair, I was stunned. This was the start of the rollercoaster journey. Having questions vaguely answered at a consultant appointment and being led to believe something may not be the case when in fact it was definitely the case was not a good experience. It turned out that this would be quite a common occurrence throughout my journey and seems to be the experience of some others also.

I wanted all the facts, I did not want to be drip fed information at the decision of a consultant who knew nothing about me and I found this very frustrating. Whatever the protocol is, there are different personality types who handle traumatic news in different ways. I wanted to prepare myself for the journey that I had started and as a single working mother it was important to me that I could organize things for my child. I did find that the consultants and Macmillan support who came to understand my personality made a great effort to help me by providing as much information as possible and things became easier. I encourage anyone to find the right support as early as possible after diagnosis.

When you do reach this stage of discussion with your oncologist you will be advised if chemotherapy will be part of your possible treatment. This day will be imprinted on my memory forever, along with many others.

I was fortunate enough that there was a wig service offered through my local hospital. I was not advised of this until the very last minute just before the treatment started.

By this time I had already visited a hairdresser experienced with chemotherapy patients, and I had purchased a wig. This was an expensive process, one I could have done to avoid at this point as money became another issue when I was unable to continue working throughout the treatment.

If I had realized there was a local wig service for cancer patients I could have prepared better for my hair loss, the fact that I was given this information just before chemotherapy started was not soon enough.

I decided to visit the hospital's wig provider as soon as I was given their contact details just to see what was offered. I would suggest asking for this information before chemotherapy starts to give you time to purchase the necessary headwear and avoid the last minute rush and stress. The wigs were fabulous; a whole range of colours, lengths, styles, and other headwear was available too. This was a huge relief and even caused excitement for the first time since diagnosis. I actually had fun at this point trying on different styles until I found exactly what I was looking for, a wig that made me look like me again, perfect.

It is also really useful to be able to try on different styles as you may want a new style, or to get as close as possible to your current look.

It is a must to purchase a pack with a wig brush, shampoo, wig sprays, and a wig stand. Make sure the wig stand is not polystyrene but plastic. The plastic wig stand allows the wig to dry after washing whereas the polystyrene wig stand absorbs water and is not useful for drying a wig at all.

It is really easy to wash a wig and the full instructions are provided with your purchase usually, or ask for them at this time.

It is helpful to purchase, or ask your hairdresser, for a stocking cap to wear under the wig initially. This stops any remaining hair catching or rubbing on the scalp which can cause soreness and make the wigs very uncomfortable.

If you do find the wig makes your scalp sore in places try putting a small amount of Vaseline on the sore parts of your scalp before putting on your wig cap and then your wig.

Certain hospitals will have charities available that offer wig banks. These are donated wigs that patients no longer need and are usually available for a nominal donation.

Hair can start to fall out just a few weeks after chemotherapy starts, usually by the second or third cycle, everyone is different; there is no set time frame for this.

People with long hair are generally advised to cut it shorter before treatment starts. I didn't opt to do this as I couldn't bear to part with my long hair and foolishly hoped I would be an exception to the rule and my hair would stay intact. Soon after treatment started however my hairdresser cut my hair into a crop to wear under my wig, at this point my hair had become quite thin and it was time to start wearing a wig. After being uncomfortable for a while and after talking to a wonderful nurse I took the plunge to shave off what was left of my hair. It felt better to do this and as though I had brought some kind of control back to a life that felt completely out of my control.

Wearing a wig is a personal choice and many people feel it isn't right for them. It is perfectly fine not to choose to wear a wig when you lose your hair and this is purely each individual's choice.

During my treatment, I met many different types of people. Some wouldn't have entertained a wig and others wouldn't leave the house without it. Do exactly what feels right for you, which goes without saying.

At the time of writing this, there is also a service at some hospitals of a cold cap. This is placed on the head during the first administration of chemotherapy. This could possibly help prevent hair loss. The hospital I received treatment at advised this would not work and could be quite painful therefore I did not choose to try this. Chatting to various people who did try the cold cap, I did not actually find anyone it worked for. By all means try it but it does not seem to have been perfected as of yet. This isn't to say that there might be something in the future which could help towards preventing hair loss.

Checklist

1. Check with the hospital well in advance of

chemotherapy for wig companies.
2. Check with the hospital to see if they have a wig bank service.
3. Purchase a wig pack with stand for drying, brush and shampoo.

TIP 2
HATS

During hair loss and until your hair grows back it is really useful to purchase a soft hat, which is simply a soft cotton hat that fits comfortably around your head. This can be purchased from wig providers or there are various internet sites which offer these for people with hair loss. Sometimes they are called a sleep cap, made from very soft cotton to keep the head cool in the summer months but also provide warmth in bed if the head feels cold. I purchased a really soft, black hat to wear during the day when I was at home. I also wore this in bed at night as my head felt cold and strange without my usual long hair.

I used to keep it in my bag during outings too. If I was visiting someone and wanted to take my wig off for a while, I would simply pop the hat on which felt comfier and actually looked quite good.

My chemotherapy treatment occurred during the summer months and the wig did become quite itchy and hot sometimes. I enjoyed being able to wear a soft hat instead.

I also purchased a couple of beautiful scarves which were attached to soft caps. After much assistance from friends looking for pretty scarves, I came across just what I was looking for through the internet. As the scarves were attached to a soft hat they fitted well and looked attractive. They even came with a scrunchy tie for different styles! I bought a few to wear with different outfits which helped brighten the situation.

I also purchased a long hairpiece which I sewed into a pretty scarf so that I could wear the scarf and have the hair as well. This meant I didn't have to wear a wig on my scalp during the warm summer months and I appeared to be wearing a scarf with hair flowing out from it giving the impression of a full head of hair!

Just a note also that when my hair started to fall out my head did hurt. I didn't imagine it would hurt to lose my hair, but it did. It wasn't a huge pain just an uncomfortable ache and it is quite a normal part of the process.

Checklist

1. Purchase a soft hat to sleep in.
2. Purchase any scarves or hats for days you prefer not to wear a wig.

TIP 3
GET OUT OF THE HOUSE

During any treatment always make the effort to get out of the house by early afternoon every day.

It may be the case that you have to give up work for a while and certain days will be spent in bed. Even during these days do your best to get outside even if it's just to sit in the garden or take a short stroll, energy permitting.

If you are able to continue working at times throughout your treatment then this tip does not apply as much.

If your treatment has the effect where you are not doing your normal routine, which is what happened to me, then getting out of the house is a major accomplishment and lifts the spirits.

It is very easy not to do this and I highly recommend making the effort, it is very worthwhile. It can be a very lonely time and going outside, even just for a minute can make all the difference to your feeling of well being.

One of the problems of breast cancer treatment is the feeling of being isolated and cut off from everything and everyone, going outside and changing the scenery for a while can be very therapeutic at such a challenging time.

TIP 4
SUPPORT TEAM

Line up a team of friends, family, co-workers, your children's (if you have them) friends' parents, anyone who can help during your treatment. Plan this help until 4-6 weeks (at least) after your last treatment as recovery can take a while when treatment has finished.

This is one of the things I found was not relayed by the medical staff or I just couldn't accept it if I was advised at the time, which is most likely the case. I kept trying to go back to work and was desperate to get back on track but didn't have the energy or capability. It actually took until a year after radiotherapy treatment for me to be able to work again full time in addition to other responsibilities as a single mother. I didn't expect this at all and felt if I had been prepared could have had more help and handled it in a better way.

During illness many people don't know what the patient needs. Communicate with your support network and let them know what you would like help with.

It may not be very helpful for a friend or family member to visit for a cup of tea when you have no energy, although they are trying to help by doing this. It could be draining to even have visitors after a certain amount of treatment as just holding a conversation could be tiring.

It could, however, be very helpful for a friend or family member to visit to bring you groceries or clean your kitchen. They will not be sure what you need so it is up to you to let them know how they could be really helpful.

I found that people were desperate to help but did not know what to say or do for the best; it was up to me to help them with this.

If you don't have any family close by or anyone you feel you could ask for help, the hospital may have support groups and services which can do small errands for you or look after children to give you a break. This is not a time to be too proud to ask for help and take everything onto your own shoulders. Many of us are not used to asking for help. We are used to juggling all the daily tasks ourselves, however, this is the time when you need to change that and find as much support as you possibly can.

TIP 5
COUNSELLING

It may be possible to have the support of counselling where your treatment is taking place. This could also be arranged through your GP.

There are many feelings that are associated with a cancer diagnosis and it can be very worthwhile to discuss this with someone who isn't related to you or who already knows you.

Professional counsellors can make all the difference to your spirit and feeling of well being during the trials and tribulations of cancer treatment.

It could also be useful for close family members who are finding your diagnosis difficult to deal with to seek help with counselling. It will affect everyone around you and it is vitally important to recognise if things are becoming overwhelming.

There is so much help and support available that you don't have to deal with the situation alone.

I would highly recommend counselling.

TIP 6
WEBSITES

The natural reaction for many people when told they have breast cancer is to go straight to the internet and start looking up facts.

It really is advisable to only look at official websites such as Cancer Research, Macmillan or other official cancer websites. There is so much information on the internet, however, much of it will not apply to you and could be very distressing indeed.

I knew to be careful with the internet after my previous experience with a family member and cancer. At that time I read reports, facts, saw photographs and read stories that were so upsetting they didn't help me or my family at all. Many internet sites may not be checked or relevant to your situation and therefore can be quite misleading.

By all means, use the internet to research your situation but use it wisely. Stay away from non official sites or blogs for breast cancer that could make your emotional situation worse.

You may find friends or family go straight to the internet and start calling with advice which could be completely irrelevant and unfounded. Remember, people are trying to help you but don't take all of this to heart, there are good official websites that give you direct support.

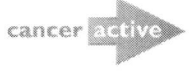 A valuable website I was directed to, almost a year after my treatment finished is www.canceractive.com. I was recommended to check the information on the site through a business contact. I also had a two hour discussion with the author Chris Woollams at a time when I had to make a very difficult decision regarding treatment and was researching support available. Although it is only yourself who can make a decision regarding treatment it helps to be as informed as possible. The website, books and advice I received were invaluable. Again, I was grateful to have found such an informative site and only wished I had discovered it sooner than I did.

TIP 7
BREAST CARE NURSE

The breast care nurse allocated to me turned out to be an invaluable support, advocate and much more over the course of three years and counting. It may be the case that you do have contact with a breast care nurse immediately after your diagnosis; hopefully this service will be available to you. This can also be found through the Macmillan website in the UK.

The Macmillan breast care nurses can be very helpful. They are available for any kind of support you may need and are there for you when you have questions, concerns or need someone to talk to.

I found their care and understanding vital to me when faced with such an unknown. It made the process easier to deal with knowing there was support available.

I hesitated at first to call them if I needed help. I soon realised having someone to answer questions and offer support was indeed a great help.

As they are used to dealing with the front line on a daily basis they had the knowledge of various side effects, an understanding of ever changing emotions and traumas of cancer treatment that I didn't always find with a consultant not exposed to these problems on a daily basis.

I also received help from my nurse when I experienced a serious malfunction in the hospital service and I was refused an examination of a new lump in my breast. I insisted on an examination and the hospital denied my request, an argument started and it very quickly went from bad to worse. Luckily, my breast care nurse was located and was able to assist with making sure I had an examination that day.

My breast care nurse also organized an appointment with my oncologist after being seen by an inexperienced registrar who was giving me incorrect information. I strongly advise if you have questions that are unanswered, even the smallest thing could make a huge difference, ask to see another specialist and don't take no for an answer.

I now donate to Macmillan every month and hope many people benefit from their care, as I have had the privilege of doing.

TIP 8
HOSPITAL APPOINTMENTS

Before your consultant appointment for oncology, radiology or surgery you may pick up a number of leaflets available which cover these subjects. These should be available at the hospital or clinic you are visiting.

Write down any questions you have before your appointment. Make sure you ask all of these questions during your appointment, do not be rushed. If you are unsure of anything at all keep asking.

It is very easy during an appointment to become emotionally upset or feel overwhelmed and forget any questions you might have wanted to ask. This is your opportunity to find out as much as possible about facts you want to know.

I would also advise taking a close friend or family member to appointments with you so that they can ask anything you may not have thought of but which could be very relevant to you.

If any of your questions are not answered to your satisfaction, keep asking, do not give up. If necessary, ask for another consultant, if you do not feel confident with the responses you are getting.

If you are denied answers then file a complaint, this is your life in the balance and you need to make sure you take responsibility for it. If your gut feeling is telling you something then you most definitely need to ask more questions and make sure you are given the answers you deserve.

Unfortunately, I did experience difficulty at certain times and as this was an emotional time already it took the strength of a giant to obtain the answers I needed. I had terrible side effects to a particular drug I was prescribed for 5 years and it took, a very painful 14 months, of seeing various specialists and filing a complaint for my situation to be taken seriously.

I had to endure these side effects which caused a whole host of problems when there were possibly other options I could try. Shocking as it sounds this is a fact, it happened to me and it can easily happen to anyone else.

If you are not happy with the outcome of an appointment then follow it up with the relevant people. There can be flaws in any excellent medical system and whilst these are under constant review it can only help other patients if you speak up for yourself. I am sure there are many women out there who don't have the courage to do this which is why it is a very good idea to take a strong friend with you to appointments.

I would also like to add that I had many great experiences from the medical profession during my treatment and this was generally the case. Even when I did receive less than acceptable treatment there was always an individual who came to the rescue on my behalf.

I learned a valuable tip during my hospital appointments which could sometimes mean long hours in a depressing oncology waiting room. Delays of up to a few hours sometimes ensued depending on the patients at the time so I decided to ask if it would be a possibility, after checking in at the reception, if I could go to the hospital café or oncology support room for a drink. The response was very encouraging as there was an understanding for the need of light relief during such difficult appointments. As long as the hospital knew I was present they would give me a time frame to check back in as they could advise if there was a delay or not.

On the days there was a delay (a common occurrence of hours sometimes) it was wonderful to be able to walk around, get some fresh air or simply sit in a nicer lounge or café as opposed to a very emotionally draining waiting area.

Obviously, it is of the utmost importance that you check back in at certain intervals as you wouldn't want to miss your appointment or delay someone else's. Each hospital will be different but it may be an option.

This made a great difference to my hospital appointments. I would highly recommend taking motivational CD's or music to your appointments also, play whatever music or CD's make you feel on top of the world. Most people have a mobile phone that has this facility so all you need is a pair of headphones and you're all set.

This puts you in a frame of mind where it is much easier to get through appointments and will change what could be quite a difficult day into a much better one.

The following may or may not apply to your situation. If the hospital you visit has a fee for parking check with their parking warden and find out if you can be provided with a notice to place in your car for free parking for the duration of your treatment.

It was stressful, with so many hospital visits, to find the parking fee required several times a week and I stumbled across help accidentally when I ran out of change for the parking machine.

I was given a notice which said I was entitled to free parking as I was an oncology patient on treatment. This was incredibly useful to have.

If I had not asked the warden when I could not find any change for the parking machine I would never have known this and any alleviation of stress was a huge help.

Checklist

1. Write a list of questions prior to any appointments and take a pen and paper with you to make any notes.
2. Take a friend or family member who may think of relevant questions you may have missed and for support.
3. Arrange transport you may need and make sure you are aware of the parking available if applicable.
4. Take light reading material, music or motivational CD's with you.

TIP 9
CHEMOTHERAPY

When chemotherapy starts you will be advised to keep checking your temperature and to avoid people with colds or any other illness. If you start to suffer with a high temperature or become ill it could mean a hospital stay.

This is due to a suppressed immune system during the treatment.

Take this advice seriously. I did not take it as seriously as I should have and directly involved myself with a family member who was not well during one of the few days out I had during the treatment. It resulted in a chest infection for me which was difficult to deal with on top of my treatment.

It is not always easy to avoid illness; however, the risk can be reduced by shopping at quieter times or just avoiding anyone you know who isn't particularly feeling well.

It is a really good idea to take a friend or family member with you to your chemotherapy appointments, even though you may think you don't need to. I did try it both with and without support and both times I decided to go to my chemotherapy appointments alone they were postponed due to a low white blood cell count. I genuinely believe this was a good thing as I was already regretting the decision of going alone when I started the appointment. It is much better to have someone else to chat with to take your mind off things.

It can be a nerve wracking experience and it certainly helps to have someone there to support you. After the first treatment you will know yourself whether or not you prefer to go alone.

I would also highly recommend taking flavoured boiled sweets to chemotherapy appointments. I didn't learn this until my sixth treatment and it made such a difference to the metallic taste I immediately experienced when the treatment started. Such a small thing was a big help.

There can be many side effects to chemotherapy and anti-sickness medication issued at the same time. If you do suffer from any side effects after your first cycle let the hospital know. There are alternative anti-sickness medications available which may not have such severe side effects. There is no need to suffer in silence and just assume this is part of the treatment, which definitely doesn't have to be the case.

Chemotherapy knocked me off my feet until the last week just before the next cycle. I made sure I planned whatever I needed to do in the three week cycle on the last week and just before my next treatment.

It really was a case of fitting in as much as I could in one week out of every three which worked as well as possible for me.

People do experience different levels of fatigue during chemotherapy but this is the general way it tends to go.

I would suggest waiting to see what your pattern is and plan accordingly.

There is a particular book that I found very helpful before chemotherapy started which pointed out some of the best foods to eat during chemotherapy treatment that would be easy to eat.

"Eating during Chemotherapy" is a book that helped me buy in the ingredients I could use before the treatment started. It has really useful recipes in it also, simple to make, which is important when you're suffering from fatigue and a general feeling of being unwell. See my book list for details.

If there are any aspects of advice you find that you are unsure of it is imperative to check with your consultant if it applies to you. There are certain foods that could contain hormones that may not actually be of benefit to you depending on the type of breast cancer diagnosed. Always let your consultant know if you change your diet or have problems eating.

Many people stop eating most foods during chemotherapy and some people have cravings for food, everyone is different.

It is also quite common to have a sore mouth as chemotherapy can leave the mouth coated and cause ulcers; this book helps deal with this and suggests easy-to-eat foods.

There are also certain foods which help with the side effects of treatment and the immune system; it is well worth educating yourself and doing as much as possible to make the situation easier.

It is also a good idea to cook any light meals you may need for the weeks you are particularly tired. They can be frozen and then just taken as required if you have no energy for cooking.

Checklist

1. Take boiled flavoured sweets to your appointments.
2. Take reading materials, music or motivational CD's.
3. It is helpful to have the support of a friend or family

member during chemotherapy appointments.
4. Cook easy to eat food in advance and freeze small meal portions to make it easier if you're tired after treatment.

TIP 10
FUNNY FILMS, RADIO AND BOOKS

After my diagnosis I stopped any kind of television, newspaper or book that could be emotionally depressing. I wasn't known to read or watch anything of this nature anyway but I made sure I kept my environment as positive as possible.

I bought quite a few funny books and found these really helpful. I took one particular book with me to the hospital before my surgery and it kept things in perspective and also kept me in high spirits, reducing my nervous apprehension. I Googled "funny books" and first on the list was a book called "The Book of Bunny Suicides" by Andy Riley. It sounded strange but had great reviews and bizarrely it is a really funny book.

I sat in the waiting room where I would be shown to my recovery room prior to breast surgery clutching "The Book of Bunny Suicides". As my sister and I leafed through the pages we found it difficult not to laugh loudly which seemed inappropriate in the sombre environment we were in.

Arrival at the hospital is usually around 6am, regardless of the time of your surgery. My surgery was changed to the last one of that day which was around 3pm so there was a lot of sitting around for me. This book was hilarious and turned what could have been a day of apprehension and worry into one of laughter. I was wheeled down to the operating room feeling relaxed and calm, I am sure that probably isn't the norm judging by everyone else's demeanor that day. I still have the book in my house and every now and then pick a page to look at and it's still funny, so thank you to Andy Riley for illustrating such a brilliant book.

I watched some great funny films over the course of my treatment. Again, these lightened the mood and really made a difference to the feeling of helplessness that appeared at times.

It was good to get family and friends involved too, keeping things on a positive level.

On the days I couldn't get out of the house I listened to the radio and even this helped to keep my spirits up and gave me a feeling of connection with the outside world, it was invaluable.

TIP 11
CHILDREN

This tip may not be applicable to you, if you do not have children. Although you may have other young family members or contact with young children, through work, for instance, and it may be helpful for that reason.

I picked up several bits of reading material from the hospital I was to be treated at. There was a section on what to tell children and also a complete book to read to a child to explain the situation.

I found the book far too much for William, my five year old and didn't feel the need to read it to him at all. I did, however, tell him rather casually while we were playing one day that mummy was going to have a treatment and that it wouldn't affect his life at all but sometimes mummy might be a bit more tired than normal.

My advice would be to tell children the basics, don't burden them with illness and keep their lives as normal as possible no matter what it takes. Obviously they will know their parent, aunt, uncle or whoever the case may be, is going through some treatment and feels ill or fatigued at times. This could be really all they need to know depending on their age.

Answer their questions honestly and briefly. If you have your own children you may want to advise their school if you need to as it may mean other people take them or collect them during your treatments and appointments. It is also helpful for the school to know in case children are affected emotionally and need help adjusting with the situation.

I kept the information I gave Will to a minimum. My chemotherapy started just before his 6th birthday. I wasn't afraid to say the words cancer but I didn't go into great detail. I answered his questions and did my utmost to keep his life normal. I did this with the help of friends and family who all helped with lifts, activities and sometimes preparing food or playing with him when I was unable to.

I explained about mummy's hair loss in a fun way and Will decided on a name for me we could use when I would become bald, which was a character in his favourite Star Wars movie, Captain Wrex, who of course has no hair. The day I decided to shave off the remainder of my hair I found a great way to introduce my new look to Will. When he arrived home from school that day I asked him to go and get two Star Wars lightsabers from his room as mummy had a surprise. He excitedly ran off and came back with his two favourite ones. I said "right are you ready to fight Captain Wrex" and took off my hat. He gasped in amazement, dropped to the floor and rolled around then jumped up and we had an amazing time, armed with our own lightsabers, play fighting at Star Wars.
I also gave Will the privilege of naming my wigs, which he found great fun and I ended up with Captain Wrex (again), Ginormica and Susan (from Star Wars and Monsters and Aliens)!

As a single parent, there were times during treatment, especially at the beginning when I would have to go and rest. Sometimes Will would play or just sit with me and quietly watch a DVD or read, this was his choice. Most of the time I did have a great support network which helped to keep his life as ordinary as possible.

Will seemed to have an instinct of when mummy couldn't play or needed to rest and was very helpful by amusing himself or just being a bit quieter.

It is always such a difficult decision when dealing with cancer and how it affects children. I am sure you will find the right way for you. If my example helps then use it or find one that suits your family in the best way you feel.

TIP 12
BREAST CANCER SUPPORT GROUPS

There are certain charities and support groups available to anyone with breast cancer.

I would stress that it is entirely your decision on whether or not you want to join one of these.

Some people find them invaluable and meet precious friends during this time. Others, don't want to be reminded of their illness and want to keep life as normal as possible.

Either way, at any point during treatment, these support groups are available.

Ask at your hospital or find them through official breast cancer websites.

TIP 13
POSITIVE MENTAL ATTITUDE

The first action I took when I got home after my diagnosis was to Google famous breast cancer survivors.

I printed out the list I found and added my name to the end. I then placed it on my office wall where I could see it every day.

Regardless of what stage you are at or what type of cancer you have it is of the utmost importance to keep a positive mental attitude.

One of the consultants I met kindly explained to me that the stage of cancer isn't necessarily the main factor in survival as it depends on how each individual reacts to the treatment plan. If this is the case or not I have no idea, all I do know is it's important to keep focused and happy.

I knew it would make a difference if I could keep my spirits as high as possible. Always a believer in positive thinking, it helped to re-enforce this by staying away from every possible negative message, as I was well aware many patients can experience depression due to the lack of control a cancer diagnosis brings.

TIP 14
WEIGHT LOSS

It may be the case that you do lose quite a bit of weight during your treatment if eating is difficult.

The hospital can provide energy drinks if you are unable to eat at times. There are also other ways to build up your strength through diet and supplements although seek specialist help where this is concerned.

I was advised to eat high fat and sugar foods during a hospital stay which went against everything I had read with regards to the cause of cancer. I do believe, in my experience, the UK hospitals are behind the times with regards to food for cancer patients. The food I was served was high in salt, sugar and dairy. There wasn't a choice of green or herbal teas and I had to meet with a nutritionist who insisted I eat the hospital food if I wanted to gain strength as I was very hesitant to eat what was offered. I questioned her in detail as I had done a great deal of research with regards to processed foods and diet. The nutritionist admitted it did not really make any sense but it was all we had to work with. I knew I had to put on weight so I ate what I was given and when I got home I went back to my healthy eating.

Much of this information can be obtained from qualified resources if you are unable to find assistance at the hospital you are treated at.

TIP 15
ALTERNATIVE THERAPIES

There are alternative remedies that can be used alongside conventional treatment which do help your feeling of well being.

It is highly recommended to try massage, reflexology, acupuncture or something similar during treatment.

There may be facilities at your hospital such as this so make sure you ask, it is not always something that is offered up front.

I was so fortunate to live near a hospital which offered patients reflexology during their treatment and it was amazing to be able to do this.

It is worth trying any alternative therapies suggested to you. It may be the case that you find something that helps you feel a little better during your treatment as I did. Just one hour a week made a difference to my treatment where I did something for me without worrying about anything else. It took a few months before I realized this and it made a real difference.

TIP 16
GET PLENTY OF REST

It may go against your normal routine to rest periodically. It is important to listen to your body and if you are feeling overtired go and have a rest.

Recovery is much quicker if you let your body rest when it needs it. The treatment can really drain you of energy so don't plan too much.

I did think that I could just scale down my life's activities a small amount. This turned out to be totally wrong for me and there were times when I chose not to do anything at all.

I learned very early in the treatment that this was going to be time out of my life if I was to help myself get through the treatment.

I found it very difficult and frustrating at times but resting did pay off and my energy returned much quicker than it probably would have done if I had ignored the signs of my body.

Listen to your body and give it the time it needs to recover during the different treatments.

TIP 17
SPOIL YOURSELF DAYS

Again, this doesn't apply to all hospitals; however, it would be possible to do something similar yourself.

During your treatment, or just after it is finished, book yourself a relaxing treat, a makeover day or something similar.

Look Good Feel Better, the international cancer support charity offer "Look Good Feel Better" days, it is worth booking one of these as it could help towards the way you feel about yourself at this time.

Make sure you pamper yourself. Cancer takes a great deal away from you and this could include your hair and energy. You deserve to do whatever it takes to feel better about yourself.

TIP 18
KEEP A DIARY

It is a good idea to write down your thoughts, feelings or side effects when the treatment starts.

It is helpful for the second chemotherapy cycle to look back and see what happened during your first one, and so on. Bear in mind that you can have different side effects during each cycle.

I also wrote down a motivational statement every time I felt overwhelmed by the treatment I was enduring. Looking back through my notepad, this statement was written down at the times I thought I couldn't handle things. It turned around my thoughts and helped me focus on the moment in time which enabled me to stop the feeling of being overwhelmed.

Other days I wrote about Will and why I needed to be there for him. I wrote about how much I loved him and how happy I was that he was part of my life.

I started writing my thoughts down at the suggestion of my GP and it was a really worthwhile process.

It also eventually led to this book which I hope will be of help to others.

TIP 19
RELAXATION TAPES, MEDITATION & SELF-HYPNOSIS

There are so many feelings that occur with a breast cancer diagnosis. It can be quite a battle with fear, lack of control, anger and overwhelming emotions.

Relaxation tapes are quite strange at first if you are used to a busy life. With practice this can be a really good way to help with different emotions and can also help if you are having difficulty sleeping.

There are many books available on meditation and this also really helped my situation, at a time when things felt as though they were spiralling completely out of control.

It may be possible to obtain tapes or meditation techniques from your counsellor, GP or hospital.

I was shocked when my counsellor suggested self hypnosis as I was having quite a problem with sleeping even though I felt completely exhausted.

I wholeheartedly dived into this possible solution and found not only was it pretty easy to do, it made a huge difference when trying to get to sleep and stopped the worrying thoughts which were streaming through my mind.

I have now implemented self hypnosis into my life and wonder why this isn't something I was taught to do from childhood. It is so relaxing to stop and clear the mind, I use it for sleeping or to re-energize, it's fabulous.

I also picked up a few other good tips with regards to sleep loss, including sticking to a suitable time to go to bed every night. Don't be tempted to read, watch t.v. or use a laptop or mobile phone when you get into bed.

Take a warm bath with lavender scent in the bathroom or put some in the bedroom. This will train your body to understand it is time for sleep and the brain will be allowed to switch off.

These are really small changes I made to what seemed to be a never ending cycle of not being able to sleep. It helped me relax and sleep much better.

TIP 20
HOW TO TELL YOUR FAMILY, FRIENDS OR COMPLETE STRANGERS

There really is no right or wrong way to do this.

You will know yourself if you want people to know about your diagnosis or not. I only told the necessary people and I found that difficult as I knew once I mentioned it then I would feel differently about that person and vice versa. Would they treat me differently, avoid me or overwhelm me with trying to fix the problem.

I experienced all of the above and would have much preferred to not have told anyone. Due to having a small child and needing help this wasn't possible and I had to let certain friends, family, school and work know what was going on.

As a person with a very busy life, a small child, hectic social and fitness activities and two different jobs including my own business, I didn't want to be the person who had to constantly rely on others. I had always coped and was always able to do everything myself, this changed so suddenly it was very difficult to accept.

I walked quietly away from the people who didn't help me emotionally during this time, at the suggestion of my counsellor. It was good advice. I didn't tell anyone I didn't have to. I found it too upsetting to talk about and usually ended up crying before I could finish the sentence.

I wanted to live as normal a life as possible and I didn't want breast cancer to define me. Saying that, if people don't know what you're going through they can't be of any help at all. This is a very difficult part of the breast cancer journey and affects people in different ways.

It's difficult for people to know the right thing to say or do. I experienced all sorts of reactions but most of them positive and helpful.

TIP 21
HOW TO DEAL WITH THE SUDDEN EMOTIONS

I couldn't believe the range of emotions I felt as soon as I was informed of my diagnosis. Anger, frustration, fear, loneliness and many other emotions hit me at various different times.

These are perfectly normal and it is ok to shout, scream, hit pillows or do whatever it takes to get it out.

It does make you feel better and as I didn't have the energy to exercise either during my treatment I did do the above instead when I needed to.

One thing I did remember learning from my own mother earlier in my life is a phrase she has passed down to me whenever anything disastrous seems to happen - "It will pass".

I started using this phrase when my family had endured Hurricane Charlie directly through the eye of the storm in Florida where we lived at the time (another story entirely) and I have used it ever since, it's very helpful.

Some days will feel like a rollercoaster of emotions where you need to cling on and wait for the calm after the storm. Cancer brings with it many different emotions. Remember this is all a normal part of the process and if it gets too much then call someone for support until it subsides.

TIP 22
RADIOTHERAPY

Radiotherapy can be a very tiring experience. Although you sometimes can't see anything visually as a result of the treatment, in most cases fatigue does play a part.

The tip I have for radiotherapy is to not purchase special, expensive creams to apply to the treated areas. Aqueous cream or similar is perfect for applying to the area on a daily basis. This is either provided by the hospital or you can purchase this cream if necessary.

Keep applying the cream even if you are not seeing any results. It is common to have a large square patch of red skin appear over the treated area. This is similar to sunburn and can be quite sore to varying degrees.

This should reduce after some time. Remember, it takes quite a while for the body to repair after radiotherapy; it may be months, not weeks, before you see an improvement.

If you have any concerns always check with the hospital.

I was given the following tip by another cancer patient just before I started my own radiation treatment and it was brilliant advice which made a real difference to me at the time.

This advice was to book the treatment first thing in the morning. My appointments had been scheduled for the middle of the day so I changed them to morning appointments. I had four weeks of daily radiation in total.

It was much better to get the appointment out of the way in the morning so I could focus on the rest of the day or just rest before my son arrived home from school and activities. It gave me a chance to do a few other things so the day wasn't consumed with each appointment.

Radiotherapy is not necessarily easy. Allow yourself as much time afterwards as you need to recover.

TIP 23
DRINK WATER

Drink water, drink water, drink water!

If drinking water isn't high on your priorities, make it the case now. Take a bottle of water everywhere you go and keep drinking it. Not necessarily a plastic bottle of water either but that is another subject and something you have to decide for yourself.

Even though this is basic nutritional information many people don't actually do it. It really is of the utmost importance during treatment and will help enormously.

Make it a habit and start immediately.

I also found Green tea a great help for my immune system and general feeling of well-being. I switched to this completely and have never looked back, I am now able to fight off colds and feel much better all round.

I drink filtered tap water, bottled water from glass bottles as much as I possibly can and plenty of green tea. Water especially helps during chemotherapy – a great tip I picked up from a hospital nurse, the same nurse who gave me the courage to shave off my remaining hair when it started falling out.

TIP 24
BE GRATEFUL

Every morning, get out a pad and pen and make a list of what you are grateful for.

It might just be something like waking up and experiencing a new day, being grateful for the love of a child, hot water, heating if it's cold outside, friends, family or a pet, the blue sky, are you getting the picture?

It will make a difference to your day if you can remember all of these things. Add to the list during the day and the next day start again.

It will surprise you how many things there are to be grateful for when it seems as though your whole world has been turned upside down.

Being grateful is not something we practice on a daily basis usually. When you change this habit, things suddenly become a great deal better; a small exercise with large consequences.

TIP 25
FINANCIAL CHALLENGES

It might be difficult to get to work during your treatment and for a while afterwards.

Financially, there could be help available. Check with your employer or the hospital if you're self employed.

Critical illness insurance could prove very useful at this time too if you already have this.

Make sure for any trips you are planning to check the travel insurance for adequate coverage. My experience was that travel insurance was very expensive so I chose to travel without cancer coverage as I felt well enough not to need this anyway.

It seemed to me that the benefit of the holiday far outweighed worrying about travel insurance and after chatting with the hospital it certainly doesn't deter other cancer sufferers from travelling either. Every aspect of travel insurance was covered except I now have a clause that if anything medical happens, breast cancer related, this wouldn't be covered.

Again, this is a personal decision for each person and not one anyone else can make for you.

During my treatment I cut down on every expense I could

possibly think of and kept bills to a minimum. This included calling the mortgage bank and changing my mortgage to a longer term as they would not agree to an interest only mortgage as a temporary measure. This lowered the payment which helped when I could not work as much as I wanted to. I stopped any service which was a luxury, worked minimum hours when I could and got through what was an incredibly financially challenging time.

Financial pressure is not a burden you need when dealing with a breast cancer diagnosis. There are many ways of easing this so don't be afraid to call mortgage companies, banks etc for assistance.

TIP 26
YOUR SPOUSE/PARTNER

There may be helpful support books that you are able to pick up from the hospital with regards to your partner.

A cancer diagnosis does affect your partner and I did read the same thing several times when I was looking for help in this area.

The main theme seemed to be that it will either bring you closer together or have the opposite affect if your relationship isn't already a strong, loving one.

If you are struggling in this area I would seek help straight away.

It could be difficult for a partner to deal with the changes a cancer diagnosis brings and it may be useful for them to seek additional help.

The main tip I have in this area is to not make hasty decisions during a stressful time and to make sure you seek help if you feel it is needed.

TIP 27
HOSPITAL STAYS DURING TREATMENT

If you do pick up an infection during your treatment it may entail a hospital stay.

I managed to get through seven months of treatment before I experienced a chest infection which meant I was admitted to the hospital.

I didn't know this was going to happen so was admitted with nothing but the clothes I was wearing. I was feeling terribly unwell for several days over Christmas and although I had asked a nurse about it before the holiday break I wasn't taken seriously at that point. During the journey to the hospital for my last day of radiation treatment I took a turn for the worse and was finding it difficult to breathe. As I arrived at the hospital I managed to shuffle through the main entrance and signalled to someone at the reception desk that I needed help before collapsing on the floor.

I was struggling to breathe and was helped to a chair. I grabbed my wig and threw it on the table and started to remove my clothes as somehow in my mind this would make breathing easier. It took what seemed hours but what was probably just minutes for a doctor to come to me. I was wheeled to a room and was given oxygen and steroids. A while later I was sent to my last radiation appointment, I was still fighting to breathe and was terrified, I knew something was seriously wrong yet felt helpless as I was too weak to get this point across to anyone. As I waited in the corridor for my turn in the radiation room I could barely move. Tears streamed down my face, I couldn't get enough breath to speak and had to fight with every ounce of energy I had to get through it. A young nurse noticed this was serious and I feel as though she was my guardian angel. She brought me some more oxygen and slowly wheeled me out of the corridor. I was admitted to the hospital and an x-ray showed I had a chest infection. This was my lowest point of my breast cancer journey in every sense.

I quickly asked my family to bring a few things to the hospital including two things I knew would make my hospital stay easier.

These were foam ear plugs and my mobile phone which had all of my music and motivational tapes stored on it. The ear plugs meant I could sleep in peace and the phone meant I could escape mentally and improve my sense of well being when I could barely even walk at the time.

I made a goal for myself to leave the hospital by New Years Eve; I didn't have a clue how I was going to achieve this I just knew I had to do it. Feeling marginally better and after five days I was dressed and waiting on my bed to be discharged first thing on the morning of 31st December 2011. I insisted I was well enough to leave and after sitting there for hours I was finally discharged in the late afternoon. A doctor never came to see me on that day and I was very relieved of this as I just wanted to get home to spend the evening in my own bed.

I fulfilled my goal of being at home and spent New Year's Eve in bed that year, I felt dreadfully ill but so relieved I was home and on the road to recovery I hoped.

Checklist

Take to the hospital:

- Night attire and day attire
- Toiletries
- Ear plugs
- Earphones
- Music, meditation CD's, motivational CD's
- Diary to make notes and pen
- Mobile phone
- Tablet and mobile broadband– not all hospitals have internet access
- DVD's
- Books
- Charger

TIP 28
SURGERY

My main tip if you are undergoing breast cancer surgery is to take a very loose fitting t-shirt or vest style t-shirt to wear after the surgery.

The breast area can be quite sore afterwards and tight fitting night attire or day attire would be extremely uncomfortable.

I also took a couple of very humorous books with me to the hospital. I purposely opted for the upbeat outlook and was helped along by the books I took with me.

It may also help to take a friend or family member with you. If they are a happy, positive minded person it will help, otherwise leave them at home!

I envisaged waking up from the surgery cancer free, well and without complications.

I focused on this all day as I was the last to be taken down for the surgery.

I have used this technique my whole life whenever I am faced with a difficulty.

My fear of flying is instantly cured by imagining myself at my destination, happy and smiling. I use this in many situations.

Needless to say I checked out of hospital at 9pm the day of my surgery and was soon at home relaxing without any problems at all even though I was the last person to have surgery that day. As an avid reader of motivational books, these are tips you will read often.

TIP 29
DECISIONS

After diagnosis, and constantly along the way, there are decisions to be made and the options will be discussed with you.

If you have several options and find it difficult to know what to do for the best this can be a very stressful time.

I found it helpful to ask the consultant what path they would take if they were in my shoes and had to make the decision for themselves. They are the ones dealing with breast cancer on a daily basis and know the in's and out's of each treatment.

They can also give you a true insight into the pro's and con's, the statistics and although they wouldn't make the decision for you, it is helpful to know what they would do under the circumstances.

TIP 30
WHEN THE TREATMENT STOPS

I was informed to be prepared for a feeling of depression when the treatment finished. I was determined this would not be my reaction and I wasn't prepared when it happened to me.

After visiting the hospital several times a week for months on end, the sudden abrupt finish of the treatment with only an annual checkup seemed daunting.

I missed being able to be around people who understood what I was going through and the environment where I felt I was fighting cancer.

I was so fatigued from all the treatment I could not get back to my normal life but I also wasn't able to continue my old life of hospital visits and the support system it gave me. My friends and family assumed as the treatment had ended all would be fine from that point.

It felt like the opposite. This is when I also really started to deal with the emotional side of things. As long as I was having a treatment I could brush the emotions under the carpet. After treatment had finished then the emotions had to come to the surface.

As I had being warned about this I had already made an

appointment with a counsellor and this was an invaluable part of my emotional journey. The real feeling of depression only lasted a week or so. I was then able to slowly pick up my life and started to very gently try normal things again.

I started slowly with just a short walk, playing with my son, re-sorting my home office, decorating and clearing clutter from my house and cooking small meals. There was quite a process to starting to feel better again.

I would advise anyone to take small steps and try not to overdo things after treatment. Depending on which treatment you have it can still be working on your body months after the actual physical treatment has finished.

This takes energy for the body to deal with it.

I was advised not to book a holiday for at least 8 weeks after the end of treatment, this was really good advice. I had a short UK break with my son around this time and travelled on a holiday overseas 9 months after my treatment finished. This was about the time I started to feel I could possibly cope with a long trip. It was fantastic and felt like a real achievement.

I was also advised by another person I met briefly who had gone through breast cancer treatment, to return to work only when I felt ready. I didn't really understand this at the time but I did find that I had varying emotions and a struggle with confidence which was so alien to me. I did small activities to build my confidence on a daily basis including going into a busy shop with my new, very short hair, making phone calls or arranging to meet people who hadn't known what I was going through.

I slowly put myself back into society and it really helped to focus on building my confidence back up to a level I was used to.

TIP 31
HOW TO GET BACK TO NORMAL

After such a life changing experience, I know life will never be as it was. Facing such physical and emotional challenges has had an effect on me in many ways.

I found after suffering from fatigue from all the treatment, one of the best ways to increase energy is to exercise.

Whether it's a walk, bike ride or joining a gym that you prefer, it is a great idea to seek the help of a professional rehabilitation specialist.

I was lucky enough to be situated in a part of the country which offered a 12 week programme with a personal trainer. This was a new scheme being offered in the area I lived. I had attempted to get back to the gym but couldn't cope very well and wasn't sure how much I could exercise.

The personal trainer put me on a one-to-one basis which focused on my short term goals (to get fitter and stronger). It took around 9 weeks for me to notice a difference with my energy levels and emotional improvement. I was able to get back to work on a part-time basis.

I started to find the energy for friends and family again, something I had been severely lacking. The smallest of tasks which seemed so difficult became easier as the weeks went by.

Without the dedication with the personal trainer I doubt very much I would have managed to improve in such a way.

I had been struggling for 6 months after the treatment finished. This gave me a whole new lease of life and I was even able to take a trip abroad with my son, a valuable holiday we both desperately needed.

TIP 32
TAMOXIFEN AND ENDOCRINE TREATMENT

I considered myself very lucky to get to the end of surgery, chemotherapy and radiotherapy treatment and was desperate to get back to normal in every sense of the word.

I started Tamoxifen a week or so after radiation finished. This was probably my lowest point while suffering from a chest infection, it was harrowing. When I was discharged from the hospital I wasn't even able to get myself from the wheelchair at the side of the car, into the car itself. I was incredibly weak, in pain and terrified; the recovery from this was incredibly slow.

A couple of times I attempted to get back to the pace I was used to prior to diagnosis which included a job, a business, a young child, friends and family, it was beyond exhausting, I couldn't do it.

I also suffered from what turned out to be severe, unbearable side effects to Tamoxifen. After several attempts over a period of fourteen months trying to find out the cause of the problems I called my breast cancer nurse in total desperation.

During this time I had a mis-diagnosis from a gynaecologist and had been referred to a dermatologist. I knew something was wrong and it took over a year of re-visiting my GP and the hospital until I finally had an answer. It was exasperating; I didn't seem to be able to obtain an answer and kept finding conflicting reports from the professional field. Always being a positive, open-minded individual I would not give up until I did find a suitable solution. I was determined that my life was not going to be like this for the next 5 years.

I was advised to speak to the support counsellors at the hospital about the frustration of fatigue and other side effects, by this point I was feeling desperate at the lack of help I seemed to find. I was instructed to go straight to the hospital and talked to the counsellors for over two hours. They advised that I was clinically depressed and to immediately make an appointment to see my GP. I did this and in a day or so I was prescribed a small amount of anti-depressant. This still didn't solve the problem of the other side effects of Tamoxifen which were affecting my personal relationship, work, how I felt about myself, and I found the fatigue crippling on some days.

I knew I was not suffering from depression; I was simply in a great deal of pain and was exhausted from this. I am not a believer in anti-depressants for myself personally and felt forced into a situation to appease the medical profession. At the time it seemed to me that I was being made to feel as though I was crazy but I knew my body was suffering in an abnormal fashion.

After finally insisting on seeing my consultant surgeon who had performed my breast surgery I was given the answers I had been looking for all year long.

Tamoxifen is an endocrine drug that may be offered as part of a treatment plan mostly to patients with oestrogen positive breast cancer. Not everyone suffers from side effects and in my case the side effects were extreme. I was instructed to take a six week Tamoxifen break to see how I felt. After less than a week I was completely back to normal with no signs of fatigue or any other side effects. I had stopped taking the anti depressants against the hospitals advice (which I wouldn't of course advise anyone else to do) as I knew this was not the problem. On returning to the hospital to discuss the outcome of taking a break from Tamoxifen I had another less than satisfactory experience.

A blood test had shown that I was pre-menopausal and I was told Tamoxifen was my only option to lessen the chance of reoccurrence. I asked for a new blood test as it didn't make sense that a blood test could be accurate that was taken whilst I was taking Tamoxifen. This was a cause of argument and I had to battle with an inexperienced registrar who simply told me I had to start taking Tamoxifen again.

Another visit to the hospital was made the following week after I called and complained of the lack of help and discussion the previous week. I still wanted to discuss alternative options as I could not contemplate life back on Tamoxifen. Interestingly enough the next set of blood tests showed the opposite result, that I was in fact post-menopausal. This opened up other options for me at this point. Or so I thought...

A third test was conducted to make sure we knew the correct result and it was disappointing to find out that I was actually pre-menopausal so we were back to only the same options as before.

I filed a complaint as I had to battle and fight to find out the correct outcome with the hospital and consultants. This is not how it should be for women who are already battling or have just battled with cancer. Any woman who is not strong enough to sort out their own health may be subjected to this difficult process. I would recommend to never give up if you feel something is not correct with the advice you are given. There isn't anyone who knows your body as well as yourself. Pay attention and make sure you agree with the outcome of your hospital appointments.

TOP TIPS WHEN DEALING WITH A BREAST CANCER DIAGNOSIS

There usually is another way, make sure you are satisfied you have searched all the possible answers and covered every option.

I managed to go back and discuss alternatives with my very helpful oncologist and I was given four new options of which only two were really a possibility. If I had not gone through the months of insisting there must be an alternative to Tamoxifen I hate to think what state I might be in today.

I had filed a complaint which led to a discussion as the procedure at the hospitals in the UK had changed at this point and the combined clinics had stopped. If I had been able to have a combined clinic appointment I would possibly have avoided the 14 months of hell I suffered whilst taking Tamoxifen.

I was not taken seriously and was made to feel as though I was insane by having severe side effects from Tamoxifen. I discussed this when I filed a complaint and it was agreed a combined clinic for my follow up would have meant a much better outcome. Hopefully, things will change in the future with this regard.

Whatever drugs you find yourself having to take after a breast cancer diagnosis it is always good to research and check that this is correct for your situation. Ask questions, questions and then more questions if necessary.

Never give up.

TIP 33
AROMATASE INHIBITORS

I tried Zoladex as an alternative to Tamoxifen and suffered similar side effects, mainly crippling fatigue. After several months of enduring this I took a break from the treatment. It took a further 5 months before I felt the fatigue lifting properly. I had made the most of the treatment free time I had, it was truly wonderful to feel almost normal again after such a long road of feeling quite the opposite.

I knew the time would come where I had to make a decision to continue with a treatment or choose not to and face any consequences that may arise. I asked for another blood test at the advice of one of the brilliant breast cancer nurses and to my surprise this showed I was post-menopausal. I consulted with my oncologist and this opened up other options called aromatase inhibitors.

I admit I was terrified of taking another drug with additives and E-numbers as part of the ingredients. I had changed my diet dramatically, avoid oestrogen at all costs, and had started a natural path to prevent any further cancer. If I picked up a food item with E-numbers, stabilizers, additives etc, I would immediately put it back on the shelf. My life now consists of fresh foods, organic choices and foods that encourage health. I learned most of this by avidly reading many books on the subject. I have no idea why these preventative pills have to contain such awful ingredients it is something I do not understand, it must have some kind of adverse effect when taken over a prolonged period. A quick glance at the enclosed leaflets of possible side effects confirms this point.

I decided to start the 5 year programme on the aromatase inhibitors and to monitor any side effects along the way. After two weeks of taking the drug I felt good and had only suffered dizziness initially. I could not ignore the advice of my oncologist, if I didn't try this and the cancer returned how would I feel looking at my 9 year old son, could I know deep down that I had done my best.

Unfortunately, similar side effects began again and I decided to take another break to make a decision of how I would move forward, with or without aromatase inhibitor treatment.

TIP 34
BONE SCAN

The reason this section is coming at such a late stage is due to the fact that this is how it was for me. I was booked for a full body bone scan due to a swelling just above my chest which had been there from the beginning of my journey. Although I had it checked at that time physically it seemed to hurt sometimes and was a bit larger, I wasn't sure if this was down to paranoia but something made me ask about it again.

Before the appointment, I received a letter saying the scan didn't involve going into a tunnel like device, what a relief. I had only ever had one scan previously in my life and that was in a tunnel like device which was OK for me, not exactly fun, but I could handle it.

I arrived in the room with the scanner and yes it was correct there was only a tiny tunnel at the end of the machine which had nothing to do with my scan. The scanner was a large (hanging patio umbrella like) contraption and I was advised it wouldn't be very nice. The scan would start at my face and slowly work its way down the rest of my body. It would be placed very close to me. I thought, well that's good I can handle this easily.

I lay down on the bed and was tied at my arms and feet, a little alarming but I was advised this was so I didn't move. The scan would take just over 26 minutes. I can only describe what happened next as absolutely awful. The top of the machine, which was hanging over my head at this time, started to lower down towards my face like a large, rock solid, very thick platform. It stopped just a tiny fraction above my face and all I could see was what resembled a huge concrete slab hanging over my head. It was so close I could feel it touching my hair and I experienced an enormous feeling of claustrophobia and fright. I closed my eyes to relieve myself of this and started to meditate.

I understood I would be around 4 minutes in this position. This really was a case of mind over matter.

Now, for whatever reason, a cancer diagnosis has lessened my confidence and tough attitude that I can do anything. I was running through my meditation, counting down steps to a warm beach with waves lapping etc etc.

Breaking through this attempt at meditation were thoughts … what if the scanner breaks and crushes my head …. it isn't moving at all … I can't breathe … where has the person helping me gone … and on and on. I knew I was heading towards real panic and as much as I battled to control this, the closeness of the machine to my face was unbearable in the position I was in. I then started to think, if I call for help and no-one is there I wouldn't be able to get out and I would be stuck so I battled to pluck up the courage to shout that I couldn't breathe and was panicking.

I shouted "Hello … I'm panicking and can't breathe can you turn the machine off". A voice replied and an assistant came to me, by this time I was truly terrified for only the second time during my journey of cancer treatment. The machine was lifted slowly up and I was unstrapped from the bed. Shaking from head to toe and crying I felt so relieved. After a quick discussion with my helper and an explanation of how the machine worked I decided to attempt it again in the same way. I could have opted to have the scan in a sitting position for the part involving my face which would take longer. I had laid there for over 4 minutes which meant the machine would have been ready to start moving slowly down my body, at the pace of a snail I might add. I had almost done it, so I decided to give it another go.

I was strapped in again and asked my helper to stand by me and count down the time on my face. This was a major improvement and although extremely difficult it was a better way to get through the ordeal. If I had known what the scanner was going to do, instead of just being told it isn't very nice, I would have closed my eyes before it even started which is what helped me get through this experience the second time. I highly recommend closing your eyes as looking at such a heavy object bearing down on you is not a pleasant experience.

I then found it fascinating to see an outline of my skeleton appearing on the screen above me as the scanner crept down my body, now that the scanner was away from my face and chest it was a great relief.

I was so dazed when I left the room I forgot to take my jewellery with me which I had to remove to have the scan. Thankfully, my helper came after me with it, so another tip from me is to leave your jewellery at home, it could have been a very costly day for me had I not had such a helpful person to guide me.

TIP 35
BE PROACTIVE NOT REACTIVE

You may wonder what I mean by this. The usual protocol is to feel unwell, go to your GP, get referred to a specialist, possibly get diagnosed with a serious illness, undergo what is sometimes gruelling treatment, recover hopefully or the worst case scenario die from that illness. That is the harsh reality people are faced with every day.

I was lucky enough to live many years in a country where people are taught to be proactive about their health, something which is alien to many people I've met in the UK, but not all. We have wonderful specialists and doctors who have a vast knowledge of illness and treatment. Sometimes, however, it is left too late for these professionals to help us.

You would think it would go without saying to lead a healthy lifestyle by educating yourself on exercise, diet, stress levels and all the ingredients that can contribute to the cause of cancer. The strange thing is, many people haven't a clue what they are doing or how they have the power to possibly prevent illness.

I used to think I lived a healthy lifestyle when actually I suffered severe stress levels continually for several years, did not put exercise as a priority and was unaware that some of the foods I ate where harming me.

Take responsibility for your body and soul, look after yourself and put this first. If your health goes, that's it, there's nothing else.

If you feel something isn't right with your body, don't wait. I went to my GP, because I found a tiny lump in my breast. I left it for two weeks after I first felt it but as it was still there I knew to get it checked immediately. This probably saved my life so far. I know this is unusual as many people have an aversion to going to the doctor for whatever reason. Please don't wait; the early detection of many cancers can be the key to survival. Not all cancer has a sign it's even there but for the ones that do, don't ignore it. Put your health first before anything else.

If you are unlucky enough to be faced with cancer treatment then I can only say listen to your body along the way and question anything you're unsure of. Your life is in your hands to some extent and with the help of experts in that particular field you can make decisions that could prolong your life. If an appointment at a hospital leaves you with questions or uncertainty then go back again or call and ask. If you find this all daunting then ask a friend or relative to help you. Don't leave it to someone else; it's your body, your life and ultimately your responsibility.

If I had not questioned the problems I had with Tamoxifen I could still be on this drug today, unable to work, look after my child or live any kind of life with any quality. It took almost a year and a half to get to the bottom of the problem and a great deal of constant questioning of professionals. Do you think this was easy? I felt seriously ill at this time too, it was horrendous but I never gave up. I only have to look at my young son and I will fight and fight and fight to be well so that he can grow up with his mum. I will do everything in my power to win the battle.

Remember, the professionals dealing with illness on a daily basis cannot possibly be attached to your outcome in the same way you are. Don't leave it in others hands, take control as much as you can so you know you've done everything possible to prolong life and beat cancer. I urge you to find the strength and do whatever it takes.

FINALLY...

Every breast cancer journey is different.

Hopefully, some of these tips will make a difference either to yourself or someone you know.

It will be a journey of soul searching, new friendships, possibly the end of some old friendships, maybe a deeper meaning to life but certainly a challenge, as great as anyone will face.

My breast cancer nurse said to me after my first chemotherapy session that each person who completes breast cancer treatment should be awarded a medal when it is finished.

I couldn't agree more.

On finishing this book I have reached three years and six months since my diagnosis. I have tried Zoladex and Letrozole as an alternative to Tamoxifen with similar debilitating side effects. I am currently considering the next option.

My life has changed beyond recognition, I live happier, I love deeper and I cherish every day. I am grateful for the people I have met along the cancer journey for their help and inspiration, including medical professionals, specialists, friends, support people, Macmillan nurses and so many more. I live a life that some people will never experience due to my cancer diagnosis so I take the positive from it and am very grateful for this.

I don't know what the future holds, just like everyone else on this planet.

Stay positive, I hope you enjoy every day and laugh as much as you can even in the rough times.

SOME OF THE BOOKS THAT HELPED MY JOURNEY OF CANCER TREATMENT

There were many books that helped me during my cancer journey including cancer related and non-cancer related books.

I am a firm believer in self-development and motivational reading.

I have included a few of the ones I took tips from and still do to this day.

I hope this list is as helpful to you as it was to me:-

- The Rainbow Diet – And how it can help you beat cancer by Chris Woollams

- Everything You Need To Know To Help You Beat Cancer by Chris Woollams

Healthy Eating During Chemotherapy by Jose Van Mil

The Breast Cancer Prevention And Recovery Diet by Suzannah Oliver

Anti-Cancer A New Way Of Life by Dr David Servan Schreiber

Cancer The Full Menu by Rolf Cordon

Stress is a Choice by David Zerloss

The Strangest Secret by Earl Nightingale

Oil For Your Lamp by Lisa Hammond and BJ Gallagher

The Everything Cancer-Fighting Cookbook by Carolyn F Katzin MS CNS MNT

Cancer Can Be Cured by Father Romano Zago OFM

NOTES

NOTES

NOTES

NOTES

NOTES

Printed in Great Britain
by Amazon.co.uk, Ltd.,
Marston Gate.